FAT LOSS

LEARN THE SECRETS TO BURN FAT FAST AND BE IN THE BEST SHAPE OF YOUR LIFE, FOREVER!

TABLE OF CONTENT

CHAPTER ONE

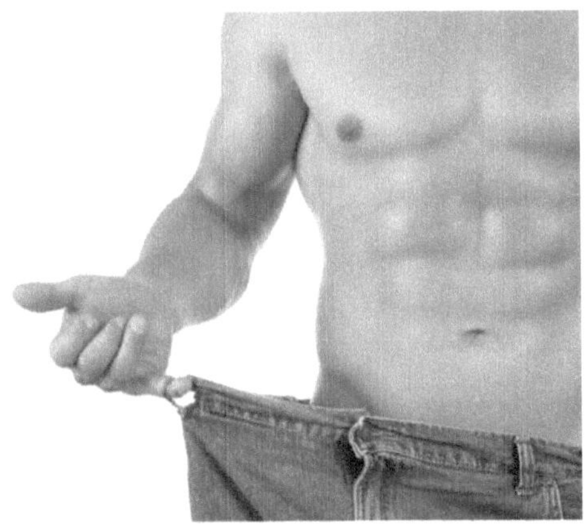

What is Fat Loss?

FAT LOSS: Fat loss is a decrease in body weight as a result of voluntary (diet, exercise) or involuntary (illness) circumstances. Most cases of Fat loss are due to the loss of body fat, but in case of extreme or severe Fat loss, proteins and other substances in the body can also be depleted. Examples of involuntary Fat loss include Fat loss associated with cancer, malabsorption (as in chronic diarrheal disease) and chronic inflammation (as in the case of rheumatoid arthritis).

Our body weight is determined by the amount of energy we consume as food and the amount of energy we spend on the day's activities. Energy is measured in calories. Metabolism is the sum of all the chemical processes in the body that sustain life. Your basal metabolic rate is the amount of calories (amount of energy) your body needs to perform the necessary functions. If your weight remains constant, it is probably a sign that you are absorbing the same amount of calories burned each day. If the weight slowly increases over time, it is likely that the caloric intake is greater than the amount of calories burned in daily activities.

If your Fat loss goals involve trying to lose 5 pounds or more than 50 pounds, the same principles determine the weight that is lost and the speed at which the Fat loss will occur. Remember the following dietary tips for a healthy and simple diet and putting them into practice can lead to Fat loss without the help of special diet programs, Fat loss programs, exercise books or medications.

Each adult controls the amount of food they eat each day. We can control our calorie consumption. To a large extent, we can also control our energy production or the amount of calories we burn every day. The amount of calories we burn every day depends on the following factors:

1) Our basal metabolic rate (BMR)

The amount of calories we burn per hour by simply living and maintaining body functions. BMR (basic metabolic rate) is defined as the minimum amount of calories your body burns if you are resting, working or lying down. This means that everyone needs a certain number of calories to stay alive. It's different for you, as it is for your children, your friends, your parents or even your siblings. These calories are the absolute minimum amount of energy your body burns and include all the involuntary activities (beyond your control) that your body makes to stay alive, such as digestion, breathing, circulation, elimination of rejection and the regulation. of body temperature.

The factors that influence your BMR include age, genetics, weight, inheritance, body fat percentage, and gender. For example, your BMR is the amount of calories your body would need to stay asleep for 24 hours in bed. The number of BMR depends on many factors, such as weight, diet and current level of activity.

BMR includes the amount of calories used for activities related to breathing, the maintenance of body temperature, the pumping of the heart, the functioning of the brain at various levels and other functions that occur in the body during your sleep. The calories burned while you is awake, on the move (including exercise) are not included in the BMR. Think of your BMR as the amount of calories needed to stay alive if you were in bed.

Your BMR slows down by about 5% every 10 years after 20 years. This is why many people do not understand why they are getting fat when they get older, but they have the same lifestyle (or the same food) in the same way. Between twenty and thirty and forty, they need to reset their BMR to reflect the changes that occur in their bodies!

Basic metabolism rates Women will naturally have a lower basal metabolic rate than men because men generally have a lower body fat percentage and a higher muscle percentage. Of course, this does not include female bodybuilders because their body fat remains below the amount of essential body fat (10-12%). With a lower percentage of body fat and a higher percentage of lean muscle mass, men need a higher metabolism to maintain this muscle.

In addition, thinner women (those whose fat percentage varies between 15 and 25%, as well as those who are active in weightlifting and bodybuilding (2 to 4 days a week) will also have a higher BMR of that of women, more sedentary, with a higher and / or overweight body fat content.

Your BMR also increases with body weight, both for men and for women. So, the more you are heavy (weight), the higher your BMR will be. At the same time, your BMR decreases with age, due to the decrease in the lean mass that often occurs in the elderly. Again, consider the fact that we noticed earlier that there was a 5% decrease in your TMB every decade after 20 years.

2) Our level of physical activity

In some people, due to genetic factors (hereditary) or other health problems, the resting metabolic rate may be slightly higher or lower than the average. Our weight also plays a role in determining the number of calories we burn at rest: the more calories you need to keep your body in its current state, the higher your weight will be. A person of 100 pounds requires less energy (food) to maintain the body weight of a person who weighs 200 pounds.

3) Lifestyle and work habits.

Lifestyle and work habits partly determine the amount of calories to be consumed each day. Someone whose work involves intense physical work will naturally burn more calories in one day than those sitting at the desk almost all day (sedentary work). For people who do not have a job that requires intense physical activity, exercise or increased physical activity can increase the amount of calories burned.

As an approximation, an average woman aged 31 to 50 living in a sedentary lifestyle needs around 1800 calories a day to maintain a normal weight. A man of the same age needs about 2,200 calories. Participating in moderate physical activity (exercising 3 to 5 days a week) requires around 200 extra calories a day. The most demanding training programs, such as those with a cardiovascular approach, can burn even more.

Fat Loss Versus Weight Loss

The words fat loss and weight loss are used interchangeably and are both often misused. But, there really is a difference between the two and there is certainly a winner. I am equally guilty of using weight loss when I really mean fat loss since weight loss sounds much better as compared to fat loss.

Here are the differences between weight loss and fat loss

Weight refers to measurement often seen in the scale- how much you weight at that particular point in time.Weight measures your body water content, bone mass density and the food you just consumed. Having that said, you get to lose a combination of muscle, fat and a lot of water weight when you lose weight. Sadly, this water weight can be easily regained.

Fat loss on the other hand refers to loss in body fat. It is said that the less body fat you have, the healthier you are. Weighing scales cannot simply show the amount of fat you lose except if you use a body caliper and even then accuracy becomes an issue here. This is because weighing scales are at times misleading regarding muscle gain as what you see as a big number may in fact mean that you have gained healthy lean muscle not fat- as muscle weighs more than fat.

Excessive body fat is extremely dangerous to your health- Obesity has been linked to deadly health conditions as a result of excessive eating and sedentary lifestyle such as diabetes, cancer and heart disease. This tells you to focus on losing body fat rather on focusing on losing that 5 extra pounds.

Another reason why it is better to lose fat than weight is because a fat cell, (or adipose cell) is much bigger in size than a lean muscle cell, which is small and compact. Having lean muscle means you will be smaller in size and fit into clothes better (no embarrassing bulges!).

Fat is much bigger in size than muscle... muscle actually weighs more than fat. I think I need to repeat that. A muscle cell weighs more than a fat cell- up to 4 times more! Let me demonstrate For example Jane weighs 145lbs (65kgs) she follows a lifestyle designed to lose body fat (like the Real Food Real Fat Loss Program), she has been exercising twice a week for 20 minutes and has lost 3 dress sizes. She jumps back on the scale and it says 140 lbs. Which she thinks strange because her friends comment and think she looks like she has lost about 25 lbs. This is what has happened... so whilst she has only lost 5 lbs on the scale- she has gained lean muscle and increased her metabolism - looking trim, toned, terrific and 3 sizes smaller! So this is why you should not get hung up on your weight!

Hopefully you are now realizing that it's better to lose body fat rather than to just focus on losing weight- both for health reasons and for size. It is best to use real food as your fat loss weapon as eating real food will fuel your body the right way & it focus's on losing body fat and increasing your metabolism. In comparison, typical weight loss diets cause you to lose muscle, which can decrease your metabolism. Now don't get me wrong if you start any healthy eating & exercise regime initially you will most likely lose some weight as well, especially in the first stages, however the continued focus should be on fat loss, which is more sustainable when following a fat loss lifestyle. Following a fat loss focused program like my real food for real fat loss program is a much better way than yo-yo weight loss. Losing fat is designed for optimum health, to increase your metabolism and keep it there- so that you will KEEP IT OFF!

CHAPTER TWO

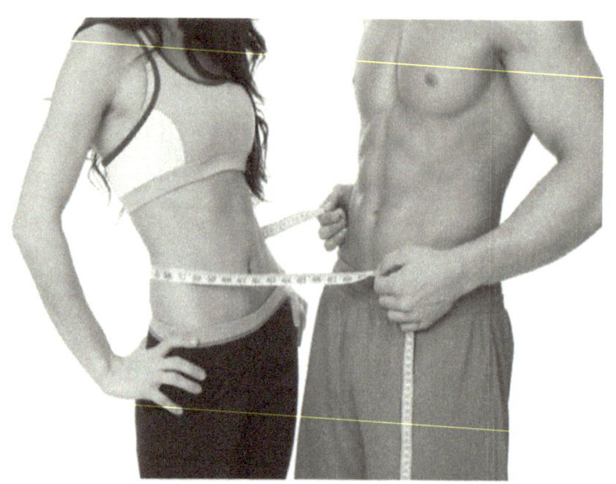

Understanding Fat Loss

There is never a time when there is a shift from one source to the other. The two are always contributing to the energy production pathways. One may be favored or dominant, but never exclusive.

Today everyone wants to be lean and mean. We all want to, not only feel good, but look good too. Everyday we work our butts off to get there and everyday we think we are one step closer. But soon a week, a month, even a year goes by and nothing has changed. What could I possible be doing wrong, you ask? Truth be known, you aren't doing anything wrong. You are doing exactly what you have been told time and time again. Unfortunately the information you have been given is based on research and studies that have nothing to do with what you want to accomplish.

"You have to work in the fat burning zone if you want to loose weight." We've all heard that before, right? But have you ever stopped to ask what exactly that means? Lets take a brief look at what this really means. Fat burning is the process where free fatty acids are used for fuel as opposed to glucose (human blood sugar). During times of very low intensity (less than 50% VO2 max) the preferred fuel is fat. About 75-80% of the energy used is supplied by fat.

This does not mean that it is the only source. It just means that there is a larger contribution of energy from fat than glucose. There is never a time when there is a shift from one source to the other. The two are always contributing to the energy production pathways. One may be favored or dominant, but never exclusive.

FAT BURNING WILL EQUATE TO FAT LOSS

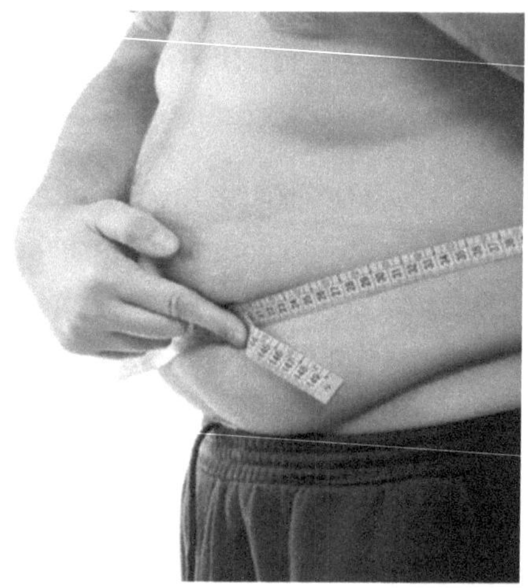

The fact of the matter is, "fat burning" has nothing to do with fat loss.[1,2,3] Fat is the preferred fuel for low intensity activity. So while you watch T.V, sit behind a desk or while you sleep! We are "burning" fat all of the time, 24 hours a day, 7 days a week.

For there to effectively be a loss of whole body fat, a negative energy balance must be maintained for a prolonged period of time. Meaning, weeks, months and years. Not minutes or hours.

This is most important point to understand and it is the one that virtually every fitness buff and expert seems to neglect.

The vast majority of us will work out for about an hour and remain sedentary for the rest of the day. That's 23 hours of little to no activity. Our workouts contribute less than 10% of our total caloric output. This is where all that research comes into play.

Lower intensity exercise for long durations may burn a bit of calories, but it does nothing to your resting metabolic rate.[5,6,9] In other words, it doesn't increase the amount of energy you expend during those other 23 hours of the day. This is the critical component of fat loss that we all seem to forget about.

DO THE MATH

Working at a heart rate of about 120 beats per min will "burn" 8 calories per min. Because of the low intensity, 80% or 6.5 calories will be coming from fat. Working at 160 beats per minute will "burn" 18 calories a min. Even if fat oxidation drops to 50% of the energy supplied, this is still 9 calories from fat every minute. So we can clearly see that if there was any validity to this "Fat burning zone" it really isn't burning all that much fat to begin with.

We can clearly see that working at a higher intensity would in fact "burn up" more fat, even if the relative contribution of fat energy is lower than at a lower intensity of exercise.

Lets make this clear, just because you burn more fat during the actual exercise, does NOT mean you will actually lose more body fat.[5] Isn't about time you asked why you haven't lost the weight you want by now?

WHAT IS EPOC?

Excess Post-exercise Oxygen Consumption. How much oxygen you consume during the other 23 hours of the day. Why is that important? Well, the amount of oxygen consumed is a very accurate way to determine how many calories your are burning. Lower intensity exercise does not create this effect.[6,9]

On the other hand both High intensity cardiovascular and weight training do. When intensities reach levels of approx 85% VO2 Max, the EPOC can last for up to 2-3 days.[11,12] You metabolism will literally be a Colorado forest fire! You can work out for shorter durations (15min) and get better results.[7,8,9]

How do you know when you've reached the right level of intensity? Well to make it simple, if you can talk to someone while your are doing it, then you aren't even close! It is uncomfortable, yes. Start slow and work your way up to it. There is no point to just spinning your wheels any longer.

And no, doing 3 sets of 12-15 will not enhance fat burning or create a more defined body. This type of weight training actually conditions muscular enzymes to become more efficient at handling lactic acid.

Lactic acid is basically a glucose molecule split in two, and being an acid, it burns. It is not, however, an indication that you are burning more fat.

DIET

As mentioned before, total fat loss comes down to burning off more calories than you take in. This is where the trainer can only educate and the trainee has to take over. Monitoring your food intake is very important to your overall fat loss goals. And if you have a high level of body fat, you will have to be more cautious on your food selections.

It is well documented that people with a greater amount of body fat, have a greater ability to store dietary fat. That's right, the human body loves its energy stores and its gets greedy!

You have to make a conscious effort to know how many calories you eat EVERY DAY. If you are working your butt off and you can't loose any fat, then you are most likely eating too much. However, do not confuse weight and fat. It is very possible to loose body fat with out seeing the scale drop. So keep that in mind. In the next article, I will show you just what food selections are good, which are bad, and I'll even tell you why!

WORKING OUT

Working out in the morning will help you maximize fat loss. You will have effectively cranked your metabolism through the roof and will be able to fuel the fat burning fire for the rest of the day. This does not mean it must be done on an empty stomach however. Low fat diets will accelerate fat loss, but a no-fat diet can be VERY dangerous.

CHAPTER THREE

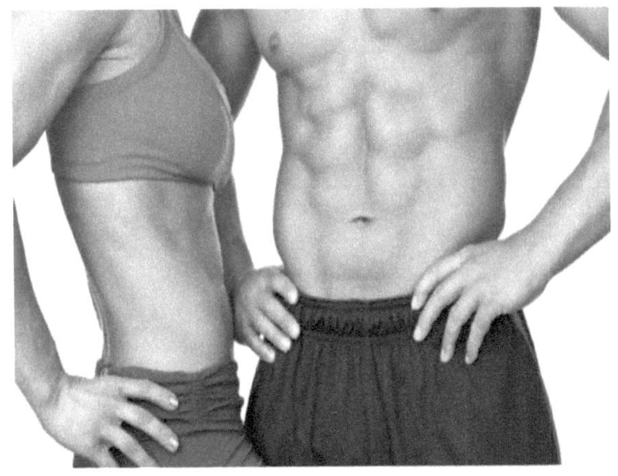

How does your body 'burn' fat?

Many of us may be considering "burning some fat" so we feel better in our bathing suits out on the beach or at the pool. What does that actually mean, though?

The normal fat cell exists primarily to store energy. The body will expand the number of fat cells and the size of fat cells to accommodate excess energy from high-calorie foods. It will even go so far as to start depositing fat cells on our muscles, liver and other organs to create space to store all this extra energy from calorie-rich diets – especially when combined with a low activity lifestyle.

Historically, fat storage worked well for humans. The energy was stored as small packages of molecules called fatty acids, which are released into the bloodstream for use as fuel by muscles and other organs when there was no food available, or when a predator was chasing us. Fat storage actually conferred a survival advantage in these situations. Those with a tendency to store fat were able to survive longer periods without food and had extra energy for hostile environments.

But when was the last time you ran from a predator? In modern times, with an overabundance of food and safe living conditions, many people have accumulated an excess storage of fat. In fact, more than one-third of the adult population in the United States is obese.

The major problem with this excess fat is that the fat cells, called adipocytes, do not function normally. They store energy at an abnormally high rate and release energy at an abnormally slow rate. What's more, these extra and enlarged fat cells produce abnormal amounts of different hormones. These hormones increase inflammation, slow down metabolism, and contribute to disease. This complicated pathological process of excess fat and dysfunction is called adiposopathy, and it makes the treatment of obesity very difficult.

A fat cell is loaded with triglycerides, or fatty deposits, and does not resemble other cells in our body. Pavel Chagochkin/Shutterstock.com

When a person begins and maintains a new exercise regimen and limits calories, the body does two things to "burn fat." First, it uses the energy stored in the fat cells to fuel new activity. Second, it stops putting away so much for storage.

The brain signals fat cells to release the energy packages, or fatty acid molecules, to the bloodstream. The muscles, lungs and heart pick up these fatty acids, break them apart, and use the energy stored in the bonds to execute their activities. The scraps that remain are discarded as part of respiration, in the outgoing carbon dioxide, or in urine. This leaves the fat cell empty and renders it useless. The cells actually have a short lifespan so when they die the body absorbs the empty cast and doesn't replace them. Over time, the body directly extracts the energy (i.e., calories) from food to the organs that need them instead of storing it first.

As a result, the body readjusts by decreasing the number and size of fat cells, which subsequently improves baseline metabolism, decreases inflammation, treats disease, and prolongs lives. If we maintain this situation over time, the body reabsorbs the extra empty fat cells and discards them as waste, leaving us leaner and healthier on multiple levels.

What foods help burn fat?

Consuming certain foods can lead to a reduction in body fat. When a person adds these fat-burning foods to the diet, they can burn fat and lose weight over time. Such fat-burning foods include eggs, nuts, and oily fish.

The term "fat-burning foods" may apply to those that produce fat loss by stimulating metabolism, reducing appetite, or reducing overall food intake. All foods stimulate metabolism. However, some types of food, such as chili peppers, might have a larger impact on metabolism than others. Eating these foods may lead to Fat loss. Certain foods, such as nuts, can also offset hunger for longer than others. Consuming these foods may help control appetite and reduce overall food intake, leading to Fat loss.

Nuts

Glass mason jars on wooden table filled with nuts, including cashews, almonds, hazelnuts, pistachios and walnuts. Regularly eating nuts can help boost energy levels and offset hunger.

Nuts are very nutritious. They are high in protein and good fats, which are both beneficial for offsetting hunger over long periods. Importantly, people can incorporate nuts into a healthful diet without gaining any weight. For example, one study from 2011, published in the Journal of Nutrition and Metabolism, found that including nuts in the diet over 12 weeks led to improvements in diet quality, without any weight gain.

Oily fish

Fish is a type of healthful food that contains vital omega-3 fatty acids. Oily fish such as salmon are particularly high in long-chain fatty acids that are difficult to find elsewhere. Fish is also high in protein. Dietary protein can offset hunger, and it is an important tool for Fat loss.

Yogurt

Yogurts can vary in their nutritional content. Plain yogurt, such as Greek-style yogurt, is the most healthful. It contains a variety of vitamins, minerals, and probiotics.

Yogurt also contains different types of protein, such as casein and whey. A study from 2014 that appears in the Nutrition Journal shows that eating high-protein yogurt can have benefits for appetite control, offsetting hunger, and lowering overall food intake.

Split peas

Split pea and lentil stew or curry with chillis. Split peas are a healthful source of energy and a versatile ingredient. Peas are high in vitamins, minerals, and fiber. They also contain complex carbohydrates, which are a good source of energy. Split peas also contain proteins that can offset hunger.

A 2011 study that appears in the Nutrition Journal explains that the protein contained within split peas has a greater impact on reducing hunger than whey protein from milk.

Eggs

Eggs are rich in vitamins, minerals, and other nutrients important to health, report the American Heart Association (AHA). They are high in cholesterol, but there is no evidence to suggest that eating cholesterol causes high cholesterol in the body. Eggs are also an excellent source of protein and can help control appetite. A study in the journal Nutrition Research found that eating eggs at breakfast had a positive impact on controlling hunger and food intake later in the day.

Chili peppers

Chili peppers contain the chemical capsaicin, which could have benefits for Fat loss. A 2012 systematic review, published in the journal Appetite, shows that capsaicin may increase fat burning and reduce appetite. These effects may help lead to Fat loss.

Coconut oil

Coconut oil contains a high level of medium-chain triglycerides. This is a specific type of fat that may have a range of health benefits.

A meta-analysis from 2015, which appeared in the Journal of the Academy of Nutrition and Dietetics, found that these medium-chain triglycerides could lead to Fat loss. However, more studies are needed to confirm the results. Many scientists believe that medium-chain triglycerides can increase energy consumption and reduce fat stores.

Green tea

Green tea has many health benefits, such as aiding Fat loss. Green tea has many health benefits, such as aiding Fat loss. Green tea is a beneficial source of antioxidants and may have several health benefits. One of these benefits includes Fat loss. A high-quality review from 2012, published in the Cochrane Database of Systematic Reviews, found that green tea consumption led to Fat loss in adults who were overweight or obese. The amount of Fat loss was small but consistently present across several different studies.

Adding fat-burning foods to the diet

In some cases, it is possible to base a meal on a fat-burning food. For example, it may consist of oily fish such as salmon with vegetables. Another option is to have eggs with whole-grain toast for breakfast.

For vegetarians and vegans, plant-based meals that are rich in protein can be a useful way to aid Fat loss. Mixing fat-burning foods such as split peas with other beneficial sources of protein is one way of doing this. Examples of this include split pea soup, or split pea dal. It may also be beneficial to choose fat-burning snacks such as nuts. Such snacks are more able to satisfy hunger and control appetite than others, such as chocolate or chips.

Certain foods can help a person burn fat and lose weight. However, it is important to remember that fat-burning foods must be part of a healthful diet overall. Also, a person must engage in regular physical activity to burn fat and lose weight.

CHAPTER FOUR

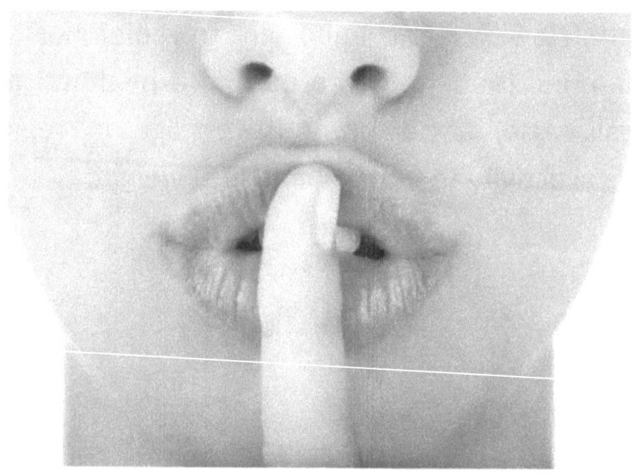

The Secret to Burning Fat Fast

If you are like most people, you probably don't have a lot of extra time throughout your day. Between work, family time, and other activities, you probably barely have enough time to sleep let alone workout. The good thing is that you aren't alone and that there are still ways that you can squeeze in an effective fat-burning workout without giving up your entire evening.

The first thing we need to discuss though is a common mistake that many people make when working out. You see, most people make the mistake of working out too slow, and as a result they never really test their body. Sure, you might tone up a bit, but unless you elevate your heart rate and start burning calories, you'll never lose those last few pounds that you need to.

One of the best ways that you can get started doing this is by implementing a cross-training routine into your weekly schedule. To do this, you just do a minute of exercise and then switch to a brand new machine. If you are at home, you can use dumbbells or tension bands to get the same effect. In some circles, they call this technique "HIIT" training, which stands for high intensity interval training. Although the name sounds complicated, it really just means that you workout at a very high intensity level for short periods of time. You can take a short break in between exercises if you need to, but the best way to burn fat is to quickly transition from one exercise to the next.

If I'm in a time crunch, I like to use this strategy at home by mixing up pushups, pull-ups, crunches, squats, lunges, and sprints. Just these few exercises alone can help you tone up and burn fat in a hurry. If you've got more time on your hands, then consider using weights or machines to get an ever better effect. You can alternative between legs and upper body, or isolate muscle groups if you prefer. There really isn't a specific way you have to organize your workouts as long as you make sure to hit each and every muscle group throughout the week.

Once you get into a routine, you will find that the pattern will help you build momentum until you get on fat burning and muscle toning roll. It might take a few weeks to start seeing results, but as long as you consistently give a high effort without resting then you will certainly notice a change for the better.

The key to burning fat is consistent effort at high intervals so that you keep your heart rate elevated for long periods of time. Don't let your body settle back down...otherwise you are mitigating the effect of your HIIT training. Keep pushing yourself harder until you start to see the results that you want. With as little as 20 minutes per day, you can implement a workout that will help you create the body you've always been after.

Secrets To Burn Fat Fast

What are the secrets to burn fat fast? Eat the proper foods, cut out the fatty foods, and exercise. Right? Wrong! Did you know that almost everything you have been taught about losing fat is wrong. If I eat better, cut down on the calories, and exercise I should lose some fat. Maybe, if your a glutton for punishment. For most of us it just will not work. We feel like were being deprived, and were starving all the time. Were definitely doomed to fail. What I am about to reveal to you will jumpstart your metabolism and literally burn fat fast. The pounds will melt away. Ok, grab a pen and write these down.

Eat

We all know what it means to eat. Eating is essential to sustaining life. Of course too much eating is why we have too much fat. Right? Wrong again! It is not that we eat too much, but that we eat too much of the wrong foods at the wrong time. Go back and read that last line a couple of times until it really sinks in. Let me explain in a little more detail so it makes sense to you. Our bodies are much like a wood burning stove. We feed the stove wood which burns and produces heat. Now, what would happen if we don't put wood into the stove? The fire goes out! It is the same with our bodies. Go on a low calorie diet and the fire goes out. In this case the fire is your metabolism. Your body goes into protect mode and the diet is doomed to fail.

Time Of Day.

What I mean here is the time of day that we eat the most amount of food. Typically breakfast is the least or non existent. Lunch picks up on the run, and dinner is from 5 pm to bedtime. This is all wrong. Our greatest energy needs begin in the morning and gradually lessen until bedtime. We should be eating our largest meal at breakfast. Less at lunch, and the least at dinner. This allows you to effectively use the greatest amount of energy or food when you need it. Skip breakfast and eating a big dinner literally forces our bodies to store fat. Change your time!

Combinations.

This is what very little of us understand. But it is vital to burn fat fast. What am I talking about? I am talking about the type of foods that we eat at the same time. Have you ever eaten a burger, fries and a shake? How did you feel afterwords.? Like a stuffed turkey headed for a nap! Why do we feel so sluggish? Because the combination of foods we ate were wrong. We mixed protein with carbohydrates and sugar. 3 different foods that take different enzymes in our stomach and intestines to process. What happens is, the food takes longer to digest. Some of the food never gets digested properly. This leaves our bodies hungry for the right nutrients. Have you ever had days where you just keep eating but never feel satisfied? Well this could be part of that problem.

Movement.

Now this is where we all need a little more help. What is the old saying "a rolling stone collects no moss." Well, "a moving body will burn fat fast!" Walking, standing, running, are all forms of movement. Our problem is we just don't do enough of it. 100 years ago fat and being overweight were not much of a problem. Most people did a lot of physical work as part of their jobs. Today we tend to be more sedentary in our jobs and lifestyle. Our life today requires most of us to push ourselves to move. But just increasing our physical movement a little will pay off by making it easier to burn fat and lose excess weight.

The Body Can Burn Fat Fast - You Just Need to Know How It Can!

Are you sick of being fat? Do you want to know what you can do to make sure you are no longer a fat slob and instead a beautiful and sexy person? There are ways to burn a lot of fast and the body can burn fat fast if you know how to get it to do this. The methods you need to know about are out there and probably are not going to be free, but they will be well worth it.

First, you are going to have to understand that if you lose too much weight too fast you are going to put yourself at risk of worse problems with your health. It takes time to burn fat off your body and you should not expect to lose more than about 2 pounds a week when you get started. However, there is a way that you can jump start your fat loss and make sure it is healthy as well.

Second, if you want to know how the body can burn fat fast you need to discover the foods that can specifically be eaten to help the body burn more fat and you need to discover the foods that will make it nearly impossible to lose weight. This is very important because if you use this secret along with exercise you can lose a lot of fat very fast and you can lose the weight you want to lose.

Last, you need to take action and stick with your plan. The biggest mistake people make when they want to lose weight is they pick a dieting program and exercise program, then they skip from one program to another over and over without ever giving the program a chance to work for them. This is something that you have to do. You have to give the program you choose a chance to work for you and that means a good 60 day commitment before you give up on it.

Burn fat fast tip

Here are some tips to burn fat fast-

1) Eat meals in small quantities throughout the day rather than having few large meals. Try and have natural and organic food, rather than eating fast food and processed food. Avoid foods that increase the glucose level. Items like sugar, pastries, desserts, white bread, polished white rice etc. should be avoided.

2) Set your fat loss goals so that you burn more calories than you consume. This can be easily calculated by using the following formula - Calories consumed minus Basal Metabolic Rate (BMR) minus Calories for Physical activities. Basal Metabolic Rate is the amount of energy your body needs while you are at rest. You can store a diet and fitness program on your cell phone or your computer and calculate the calories that you burn on a regular basis.

3) Do resistance training regularly. This will really help you to burn fat fast. Find a certified trainer who

can help you in this. Otherwise you can refer to some good book, that gives resistance training step by step. The idea here is to make sure you do the training correctly.

4) Keep yourself updated about health and nutrition facts. You can subscribe to some magazines and also enroll with some Fat loss forums. This will not only help you in keeping motivated, but also provide regular information on the latest products and services.

What Is the Best Workout to Burn Fat Fast?

For decades we've been told that the best workout to burn fat fast and lose weight is around thirty-five minutes of modest aerobic exercise (for instance running, riding a bicycle, or swimming), carried out about five times each week. In reality, many health and fitness experts still recommend this strategy.

New research results now reveal this isn't the best workout to burn fat fast. Whilst it's true that this kind of physical exercise can help you to burn off a few calories through the exercise session, you will find greater ways to plan your training so that you can fire up the metabolism to a lot higher degree and definitely burn fat fast. This will cause you to burn far more calories, both throughout and after the exercise session, and possesses a greater and more long lasting effects on your physique.

A fantastic way to increase your metabolism in this manner and consequently burn fat fast is simply by raising the intensity of the workout, while at the same time cutting down its duration. In other words, you challenge your body with a brief burst of really intense exercise, rather than settling into a lengthy, slow training. The true secret to this is the body's Resting Metabolism Rate (RMR) - the rate at which your body burns calories whilst it's regenerating. Almost all calories are burned up within the muscles, even at rest. Any time a muscle is pushed to execute an extremely intensive exercise session, it's RMR rises considerably, and it continues to burn off a lot of energy even after the training. What this means is we burn fat fast.

One of the best methods to produce this type of effect is via strength training (also referred to as resistance training). If you undertake strength training with free weights, your muscles have to defeat the opposing force of gravity in an effort to contract, and thus move the weight load. This will cause the muscle to burn plenty of energy, both through the workout, and during the regeneration process later on. Plus the fantastic thing about this really is that the regrowth process triggers an increase of lean muscle mass, which in turn allows you to burn far more energy in future exercise sessions. As your muscles grow stronger, they will grow to be dependable allies in the pursuit to burn up calories and shed weight.

Another advantage of this best workout to burn fat fast would be that the training is shorter, and for that reason easier to squeeze into a hectic lifestyle. Very intense workouts performed 2 or 3 times a week are enough to generate a solid and fast fat burning effect, and when combined with the correct nutrition approach will certainly enable you to get a trimmed and healthful body. This is the absolute best workout to burn fat fast.

How to Burn Fat Fast and Stay Healthy

Consider this fact when ever you think of losing weight, "fat is not as important as calories for controlling weight". Concerning your eating habit, you must make sure you are eating healthy monounsaturated and poly-unsaturated fats instead of saturated and Trans fat. The less, the better. Avoid eating more than 20 grams of saturated fat per day.

Strength training which means weight training in the gym or at home at least 30mins, 2 x per week as this will help you tremendously in burning fat.

Cut down on processed foods. Eat more natural foods which have little added preservatives and chemicals.

Eat more, eating well does not cause you to add more weight. Instead of the 3 square meals a day, go for 5 to 6 micro meals to keep your metabolism geared up to burn and your insulin levels steady.

Try to exercise at least 4 to 5 sessions per week, as exercising, 4-5 sessions per week will help you in getting a quicker result, and a clear difference.

Eat more protein. Your body needs protein to support the muscle it has. Make sure you are sticking with quality proteins like lean meats, fish, and poultry. Whey and Soy Proteins are also very good choices. Try as much as you can, and stay away from meats with high saturated fats.

Do something fun and always think in terms of physical activity, and always ask yourself how can I be more active today?

Control your portions by eating low energy-density foods. Foods such as vegetables and fruits have low energy density which make them less likely to be over-eaten. They are packed with nutrients such as vitamins and minerals which ensure your metabolism has the resources to do its job more efficiently.

Cardio exercise do interval training on an exercise of your choice, like running - warm-up 5mins then do 1min fast, 1 minute slow continuously for 20 minutes. AB Cirle Pro can help a lot during your exercise. See example of the AB Circle Pro from the web site below this article.

Do not cut out any one food group. Try as much as you can, and be consuming carbohydrates, protein, and fat at every meal. This will keep you balanced and fit.

Drink more Water, because water is a major player in weight control. Besides being a major part of your body, water helps flush metabolic wastes keeping your metabolism charged at all time. Water will also helps you feel fuller, helping you to eat less. You dont have to wait until you feel thirsty. Start by drinking at least a half-gallon of water everyday. Active people drink up to a gallon per day.

Eat more fiber. By consuming at least 30 grams of fiber daily, you will feel fuller than you would by not eating the fiber. Fiber also helps out your health by latching on to LDL cholesterol and flushing it out of your system. Some good sources of fiber include vegetables (which is very good for your skin), fruits, whole-grain breads, and high fiber cereals such as Kashi. To boost your fiber intake you should be eating more Oranges instead of drinking Orange Juice which contain presevertives. Oranges has less calories, more fiber and bound to make you feel more satisfied.

Eat your complex grains early in the day and then stick with the water rich carbohydrates such as fruit in the evening. This has to do with the way insulin is secreted into the bloodstream.

While eating healthy is a good start, you will never going to reach your full potential for a leaner body unless you get active and start sleeping better.

Aim to sleep well, lets asy 7-8 hours per night More or less than that can have negative effects on your health.

Stay away from fast or junk food, or at least don't eat it as often as they do contain too much calories. In fact, it is a far healthier option to cook a nice meal at home.

Eat your meals slower. It takes about 20 minutes for your body to know when you're full. If you eat too quickly, you may have eaten too much before your body knows when the limit is reached.

Eat some fish. Fish, such as salmon, it is rich in Omega-3s, which is an Essential Fatty Acid. This will help in keeping your heart healthy, and keeps the bad fat out. Fatty fish such as salmon, halibut and shellfish help reduce the size of fat cells and help out with fat loss.

Exercising in the mornings before you eat breakfast is essential, especially if you want to burn fat more effectively. Perhaps go for a mile jogging around your neighborhood, or walk the dog. Doing aerobic (fast paced) exercises after you've been fasting for 8 hours will speedily force your body to burn fat instead of calories for energy.

CHAPTER FIVE

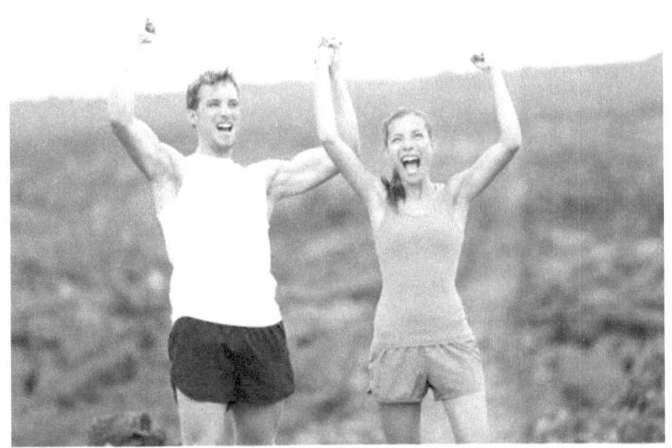

The 21 days challenge for Fat Loss

How to Lose Weight in three weeks

1. The first thing you need to address is your eating habits - losing weight is not about starvation. It's about cutting down on the processed foods, junk foods, take out and fast foods. Fact is eating more fresh foods and cooking it yourself is the best way to lose weight, long term. And without question, if you can add in plenty of fiber, protein, lean fat and whole-grain products into your meals - you will improve your diet and shrink belly fat.

2. Fat has developed a bad name, yet it is still - in moderate amounts - vital to our diets. Butter, margarine, oil and cream are all fats. Fats are categorized as saturated and unsaturated, with saturated fats - which are usually of animal origin - thought to contribute more to health problems like coronary artery disease and weight gain than unsaturated fats, which mostly originate from plants and fish. Most take away foods and junk foods are high in fat content, so it is important not to base your entire diet on this type of food. Try to replace the saturated fats with poly-unsaturated and mono-unsaturated fats.

3. Don't feel guilty - on the days where you eat too much or skip the gym, chalk it up to being human and steer yourself back on track the next day. Look at it this way- we're not perfect and there's no such thing as the perfect plan. Fat loss is about a journey where you'll have your highs and lows - but more importantly staying focused towards your end journey - shrink belly fat and improve your overall health.

4. Cut back on the diet sodas to shrink belly fat- because diet drinks, such as diet sodas and Crystal Light, are artificially sweetened, they typically contain 5 calories max per serving. So they don't

directly lead to weight gain. But guzzling these beverages all day long does lead to one potential problem - you drink less of everything else - water. So having 1 or 2 diet sodas a day is fine, but if you're downing 5 or 6 '12 ounce' bottles, that means you're limiting your intake of healthier beverages, such as tea. Best tip here is - drink water. It's simply better and calorie free!

5. The importance of exercise lies not in its degree of difficulty but in its consistency. As with diet, moderation, and balance is the key. Suddenly, starting a strenuous, complicated exercise program is almost doomed to failure. Here's how to start in a way that makes it more likely that you'll keep up the good work. Set achievable goals; a 20 minute walk three times a week may be enough to start with; set yourself harder goals once you've got going. Exercise in company; ask a friend with a similar level of fitness to come along. Work it into your daily routine; take the dog for a run, leave the car at home and walk to the shops and use the stairs instead of the lift. Vary the routine; it gets boring to run around the oval every morning. Alternate with swimming, tennis, walking or other favorite activities.

6. Don't make drastic changes overnight - With Fat loss, there are no quick fixes. Just look at gradual

improvements to your lifestyle. Overtime, you will see results that will stick.

44

21 Day Guide to Fat Loss

Monday

Tuesday

Wednesday

Thursday

Friday

Saturday

Sunday

For simplicity's sake, we'll start with Day 1 as a Monday. If you apply all of the lifestyle changes you'll find that making the correct and healthy choices is easier and more effective.

Plus, if you follow this easy to use schedule, you won't find these changes overbearing. In fact, you'll look forward to one new challenge everyday – until this new lifestyle is a habit.

Day 1 – Monday: Recruit your support partner and set your goals. Start the exercise program with Workout A. Exercise conservatively, work at your own level, and stick to our guidelines. Perform every exercise with perfect technique.

Day 2 – Eliminate all sources of liquid calories and replace these drinks with water and Green Tea. Start to enter your food intake on your personal plan sheet or time table and continue to do so for the next 7 days.

Day 3 – As you workout, visualize yourself reaching your goals. Keep a positive attitude and you will remain motivated and you will continue to make progress.

Day 4 – Make sure that you are eating 6 small meals per day rather than 2-3 large meals. Spread your protein, fiber, fruits and vegetables throughout the day to help you reduce your appetite and keep your energy levels up.

Day 5 – Clean out cupboards and prepare a healthy shopping list. Complete your 7 day food entry on your personal plan sheet or time table and review the results to help you organize your shopping list.

Day 6 – Report to a member of your support group on this day and review how your first week went. Always be accountable to your support group. This will encourage you to stick with the exercise and nutrition program.

In addition, take some time and pick an activity you really like to do (yoga, sport, martial art, dance) and make it a regular habit on Saturdays. This can be done on your own or with your social support group. images3

Day 7 – Sunday: Plan ahead for the next week and do all of your grocery shopping and meal preparation. Do some extra cooking, chop your vegetables and wash your fruit. By doing this, you will be prepared to avoid unhealthy eating situations that lead you to cheat on your plan.

Day 8 – Make sure you are doing things correctly. Hire a trainer for one session and make them a part of your support team. To help you stick to your workouts, book each exercise session like any other appointment in your daily schedule. Let nothing, except real emergencies, come between you and your workouts.

Day 9 – Today you will make an effort to eat one new fruit and one new vegetable. If you aren't already eating grapefruit, try one today and see how it helps fill you up because it contains a lot of soluble fiber called pectin. Add a new vegetable to your meal plan

Day 10 – Eliminate all sources of trans-fatty acids from your diet.

Day 11 – Review your water intake and confirm that you are consuming enough water each day to keep you hydrated and healthy, as well as using water to stay full.

Day 12 – Review your nutrition. Check the number of calories you are consuming. Are you still eating too much? Are you eating too little (less than 1500 calories) evaluate your nutrition list.

Day 13 – Check your fiber intake and make sure you meet the recommended intake (up to 35 grams per day). Eat more almonds to get fiber and keep your appetite in check.

Day 14 – Sunday: Plan, shop, & prepare for the week ahead. Make sure to include 1 new fruit and 1 new vegetable in your grocery list. Variety in your nutrition is very important, so try a new fruit today such as blackberries, blueberries, or raspberries.

Day 15 – Set a new short-term goal for your workouts, such as using a higher level on your cardio machine or performing one extra pushup per set.

Day 16 – Purchase a new cooking appliance, such as a grill or steamer to help you eat healthy, nutritious, low-fat foods in a convenient manner.

Day 17 – Try an alternative source of lean protein at dinner, such as lean beef or salmon (in case you have been eating only chicken and tuna)

Day 18 – Re-read the Turbulence Training Workout Manual and go over the nutrition section, the new workout section, and the exercise description section to double check your habits.

Day 19 – Take time and review the goals that you set. Have you met all of your short-term goals? Are you getting closer to your long-term goals? If you aren't, determine the obstacles in your way and make a plan to get around them.

Day 20 – Recruit a new member into your social support, such as a new workout partner or healthy-eating partner. This will add strength to your commitment.

Day 21 – Sunday: 30 minutes of activity. Plan, make a shopping list, shop, & prepare. Include one new source of lean protein in your shopping list.

CHAPTER SIX

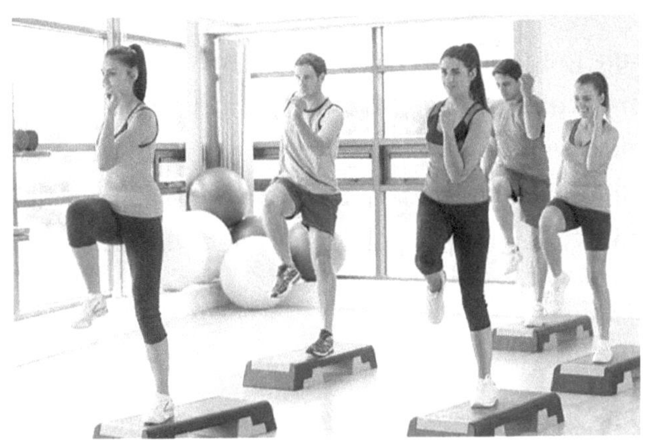

weight loss health best practices to burn belly fat

We often live a life full of junk food laden with unhealthy calories. Because we are always running away, it is impossible for most of us to manage a healthy diet. So, what do we end? Eat packaged foods or junk food at your disposal. As a result, we get an excess of fat and do not count calories that do not burn. People gain abdominal fat for many reasons, including poor nutrition, lack of exercise and stress. Improving nutrition, increasing physical activity, reducing stress and making other changes in lifestyle can help people lose abdominal fat.

1) Opt for whole grains:

whole grains mean better fibers, more nutrition and more protein and calcium. The consumption of more fiber is very useful to maintain intestinal health. In addition, it is necessary to replace the refined flour with whole grains because it is very unhealthy and can hinder digestion.

2) Burpee:

If you want to lose the gut, you must work as many muscles as possible. The burpee does just that. The explosive exercise of moving from a push-up position to a jump and then back to a push-up position affects every muscle from head to toe. In fact, a recent study by the American College of Sports Medicine revealed that 10 rapid repetitions are just as effective in increasing metabolism as a 30-second sprint. This way you can burn belly fat faster than ever.

3) Enjoy the hot organic teas:

This may include green tea, jasmine tea, cinnamon tea or other tea flavored with natural spices. Drinking hot and organic tea is very useful for losing weight because they are rich in antioxidants and contain minimal amounts of many other vitamins and minerals.

4) Mountaineer:

Think of the climber as a moving board. Make a mini crunch when you kneel explosively in your chest. However, what makes this movement so difficult is that your center has to work extraordinarily to keep your body immobile and upright every time you lift one foot off the ground.

5) Improve your sleep pattern:

Sleep is vital for the general health of people and insufficient rest can have serious consequences for well-being. The main purpose of the sleep is to allow the body to rest, heal and rejuvenate, but it can also have an impact on a person's weight. Getting enough good quality sleep is essential when someone is trying to lose weight, including abdominal fat.

6) Kettlebell Swig

The kettlebell swing could be one of the best calorie burning exercises of all time. To push the heavy iron ball, you must involve large and burning muscle groups, such as the glutes, hips and quadriceps. The explosive nature of this movement immediately increases your heart rate, but also your heart. The bell impulse on the top of the swing will try to push you forward. Therefore, it is necessary to tighten the abdominals as if you were making a table.

7) Stop smoking:

Smoking is a risk factor for increasing abdominal fat, as are many other serious health problems. Quitting smoking can significantly reduce the risk of excess fat in the abdomen and improve overall health.

8) cider vinegar:

Apple cider vinegar is an excellent natural stimulant of bile and an antacid reflux. Maintains the pH balance of the stomach so that the belly is flatter. Add a capful to half a glass of water and drink it after waking up. You can also try to cook with him. A healthy diet and an active lifestyle can help people lose abdominal fat and reduce the risk of associated problems. A slimmer waist, a healthier body and a lower risk of chronic disease start today with these tips to combat belly fat.

CHAPTER SEVEN

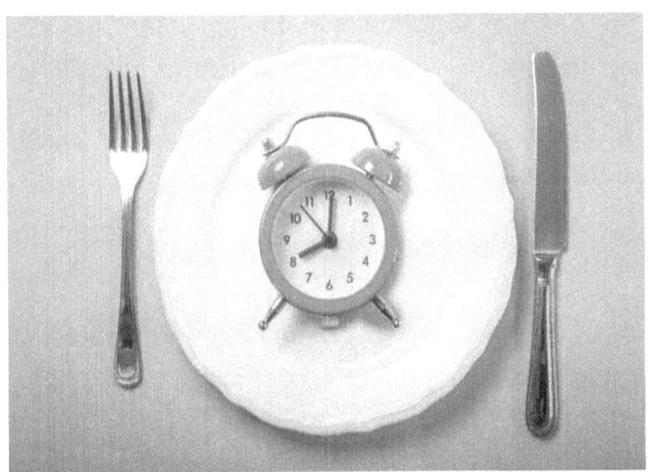

intermittent fasting

Intermittent fasting is not a diet. It is a timed approach to eating. Unlike a dietary plan that restricts where calories come from, intermittent fasting does not specify what foods a person should eat or avoid. Intermittent fasting may have some health benefits, including Fat loss, but is not suitable for everyone.

Intermittent fasting involves cycling between periods of eating and fasting. At first, people may find it difficult to eat during a short window of time each day or alternate between days of eating and not eating. This article offers tips on the best way to begin fasting, including identifying personal goals, planning meals, and establishing caloric needs.

Intermittent fasting is a popular method that people use to:

- simplify their life
- lose weight
- improve their overall health and well-being, such as minimizing the effects of aging

Though fasting is safe for most healthy, well-nourished people, it may not be appropriate for individuals who have any medical conditions. For those ready to start fasting, the following tips aim to help them make the experience as easy and successful as possible.

1. Identify personal goals

Typically, a person who starts intermittent fasting has a goal in mind. It may be to lose weight, improve overall health, or improve metabolic health. A person's ultimate goal will help them determine the most suitable fasting method and work out how many calories and nutrients they need to consume.

2. Pick the method

Intermittent fasting for Fat loss

Typically, a person should stick with one fasting method for a month or longer before trying another.

There are four potential methods that a person may try when fasting for health reasons. A person should pick the plan that suits their preferences and which they think they can stick with.

These include:

- Eat Stop Eat
- Warrior Diet
- Leangains
- Alternate Day Fasting

Typically, a person should stick with one fasting method for a month or longer to see if it works for them before trying a different method. Anyone who has a medical condition should talk to their healthcare provider before beginning any fasting method.

When deciding on a method, a person should remember that they do not need to eat a certain amount or type of food or avoid foods altogether. A person can eat what they want. However, to reach health and Fat loss goals, it is a good idea to follow a healthful, high-fiber, vegetable-rich diet during the eating periods. Binging on unhealthful foods on eating days can hinder health progress. It is also extremely important to drink lots of water or other no-calorie beverages throughout the fast days.

Eat Stop Eat

Brad Pilon developed Eat Stop Eat, which is a fasting method that involves eating nothing for 24 hours twice a week. It does not matter what days a person fasts or even when they begin. The only restriction is fasting must last for 24 hours and on non-consecutive days. People who do not eat for 24 hours will likely become very hungry. Eat Stop Eat may not be the best method for people who are unfamiliar with fasting to start with.

Warrior Diet

Ori Hofmekler is the creator of the Warrior Diet, which entails eating very little for 20 hours each day. A person fasting in this way consumes all their typical food intake in the remaining 4 hours.

Eating a whole day's worth of food in such a short time can make a person's stomach quite uncomfortable. This is the most extreme fasting method, and similarly to Eat Stop Eat, a person new to fasting may not want to start with this method.

Leangains

Martin Berkhan created Leangains for weightlifters, but it has gained popularity among other people who are interested in fasting. Unlike Eat Stop Eat and the Warrior Diet, fasting for Leangains involves much shorter periods.

For example, males who choose the Leangains method will fast for 16 hours and then eat what they want for the remaining 8 hours of the day. Females fast for 14 hours and eat what they want for the remaining 10 hours of the day. During the fast, a person must avoid eating any food but can drink as many no-calorie beverages as they like.

Alternate Day Fasting, 5:2 method

Some people fast on alternate days to improve blood sugar, cholesterol, and Fat loss. A person on the 5:2 method eats 500 to 600 calories on two non-consecutive days each week.

Some alternate-day fasting regimens add in a third day of fasting each week. For the rest of the week, a person eats only the number of calories they burn during the day. Over time, this creates a calorie deficit that allows the person to lose weight. Resources on the Eat Stop Eat, Warrior, and Leangains fasting methods are available to purchase online.

3. Figure out caloric needs

There are no dietary restrictions when fasting, but this does not mean calories do not count. People who are looking to lose weight need to create a calorie deficit for themselves — this means that they consume less energy than they use. People who are looking to gain weight need to consume more calories than they use.

There are many tools available to help a person work out their caloric needs and determine how many calories they need to consume each day to either gain or lose weight. A person could also speak to their healthcare provider or dietitian for guidance on how many calories they need.

4. Figure out a meal plan

Intermittent fasting for Fat loss meal prepare

Making a meal plan for the week may help someone who is trying to lose or gain weight. A person interested in losing or gaining weight may find it helps to plan what they are going to eat during the day or week. Meal planning does not need to be overly restrictive. It considers calorie intake and incorporating proper nutrients into the diet. Meal planning offers many benefits, such as helping a person stick to their calorie count, and ensuring they have the necessary food on hand for cooking recipes, quick meals, and snacks.

5. Make the calories count

Not all calories are the same. Although these fasting methods do not set restrictions on how many calories a person should consume when fasting, it is essential to consider the nutritional value of the food. In general, a person should aim to consume nutrient-dense food, or food with a high number of nutrients per calorie. Though a person may not have to abandon junk food entirely, they should still practice moderation and focus on more healthful options to gain the most benefits.

<u>How effective is intermittent fasting</u>

Fasting has several effects on a person's body. These effects include:

Reducing levels of insulin, which makes it easier for the body to use stored fat.

Lowering blood sugars, blood pressure, and inflammation levels.

Changing the expression of certain genes, which helps the body protect itself from disease as well as promoting longevity.

Dramatically increases human growth hormone, or HGH, which helps the body utilize body fat and grow muscle.

The body activates a healing process doctors call autophagy, which essentially means that the body digests or recycles old or damaged cell components.

Fasting dates back to ancient humans who often went hours or days between meals as obtaining food was difficult. The human body adapted to this style of eating, allowing extended periods to pass between food intake times.

Intermittent fasting recreates this forced-fasting. When a person undertakes an intermittent fast for dietary proposes, it can be very effective for Fat loss. In fact, according to one study, most people try intermittent fasting to help lose weight.

Other research backs up the claims that fasting can help a person lose weight. For example, a review of studies shows that many people who fast see a higher loss of visceral body fat and a similar to slightly less reduction in body weight compared with people who follow more traditional calorie reduction diets.

Research also shows fasting to be beneficial for the management of metabolic syndrome and diabetes, extending lifespan, protecting neuron function, and shows promise in those with digestive diseases.

Side effects

Intermittent fasting for Fat loss not advised for pregnancy. Pregnant women may be at risk from fasting and should consult a doctor before trying any program. For a healthy, well-nourished person, intermittent fasting offers very few side effects.

When a person first starts fasting, they may feel slightly physically and mentally sluggish as their body adjusts. After the adjustment, most people go back to functioning normally.

However, people with medical conditions should consult their doctor before beginning any fasting program. People particularly at risk from fasting and who may require medical supervision include:

- women who are breastfeeding
- women who are pregnant
- people who are trying to conceive

- people with diabetes
- people who have difficulty regulating sugar
- people with low blood pressure
- people on medications
- people with eating disorders
- people who are underweight

Effects on exercise

For healthy individuals, intermittent fasting should not affect their ability to exercise except during the period when the body is adjusting to the new eating schedule. After the adjustment period, a person should not feel any ill effects from fasting on their exercise routine.

Those worried about losing muscle while fasting should be sure to consume enough protein during eating periods and participate in resistance training regularly. By keeping protein intake up, a person is less likely to lose muscle mass from fasting.

Fasting is a natural part of the human life cycle. Most people have fasted unknowingly throughout their lifetimes by eating an early dinner and skipping breakfast the next day. More structured approaches may work well for some people.

However, it is important to keep in mind that although a person does not need to exclude certain foods from their diet, they should still aim to eat a balanced diet rich in protein, fiber, and vegetables. Remember to drink plenty of fluids, too.

Finally, though the average person will likely experience no or minimal side effects, people with certain medical conditions or who are taking certain medications should speak to their doctor before trying a fasting plan.

Secrets to Successful Fasting - Five Keys to Make Your Fast Work

Fasting is becoming more and more popular, both as a weight-loss diet and as a long-term healthy lifestyle choice. Many people have questions about how to set up a fasting diet. Here are five key points to get you started.

1: Choose how long your fast will be

The possibilities here are endless. However, most effective plans use a technique called intermittent fasting. This involves alternating periods of fasting and periods of normal (although healthy) eating. Perhaps the two most common methods are a 16 hour daily fast (think overnight until lunch the next day), and a 24 hour period one or two times a week. The beauty of both of these schemes is that they can be made to fit in with you and your life.

2: Drink more water

This is a simple trick that serves two purposes. Firstly, this will increase satiety (the feeling of being full), which is psychologically very important when you are not eating. Secondly, this will accelerate the cleansing effect of a fast, and allow your body to function optimally.

3: Break your fast with a healthy meal

Again the interest here is twofold. firstly, when you are getting a healthy meal in first, you are simply leaving less space to eat crap during the rest of your eating "window", which is a guaranteed method to reduce that waistline. Secondly, eating a high sugar meal immediately after fasting will drive your insulin sky-high. Spending your eating hours crashed out in a carb-induced sleep is not the best way to eat! There is one exception here. Is your first meal coincides with training, it is good to release insulin. This will help the body drive nutrients into the muscles rather than stocking them as fat.

4: Workout regularly

This should be a no-brainer, but working out and particularly weight-training should be at the heart of every diet. This gives you the opportunity to eat more while still burning fat, increases muscle-mass which in turn increases metabolic rate (meaning you burn more calories doing nothing) and will make the biggest difference to your appearance in the shortest time.

5: Follow a plan

Again, this should be fairly obvious, but the easiest way to succeed with a diet and exercise regime is to remove any choice. Don't over-think things. By following a plan, you are relying on an expert who has already thought it through. Just follow the instructions.

Seven ways to do intermittent fasting

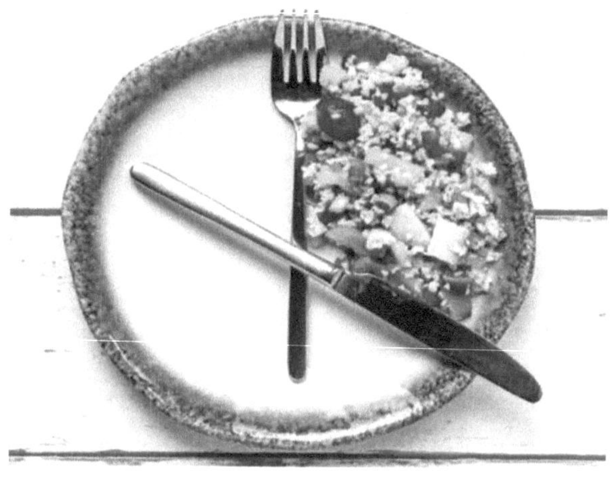

There are many different ways of intermittent fasting. The methods vary in the number of fast days and the calorie allowances. Intermittent fasting involves entirely or partially abstaining from eating for a set amount of time, before eating regularly again. Some studies suggest that this way of eating may offer benefits such as fat loss, better health, and increased longevity. Proponents claim that an intermittent fasting program is easier to maintain than traditional, calorie-controlled diets. Each person's experience of intermittent fasting is individual, and different styles will suit different people.

Seven ways to do intermittent fasting

There are various methods of intermittent fasting, and people will prefer different styles. Read on to find out about seven different ways to do intermittent fasting.

1. Fast for 12 hours a day

Empty plate on wooden table with knife and fork and alarm clock. Different styles of intermittent fasting may suit different people. The rules for this diet are simple. A person needs to decide on and adhere to a 12-hour fasting window every day. According to some researchers, fasting for 10–16 hours can cause the body to turn its fat stores into energy, which releases ketones into the bloodstream. This should encourage Fat loss.

This type of intermittent fasting plan may be a good option for beginners. This is because the fasting window is relatively small, much of the fasting occurs during sleep, and the person can consume the same number of calories each day. The easiest way to do the 12-hour fast is to include the period of sleep in the fasting window. For example, a person could choose to fast between 7 p.m. and 7 a.m. They would need to finish their dinner before 7 p.m. and wait until 7 a.m. to eat breakfast but would be asleep for much of the time in between.

2. Fasting for 16 hours

Fasting for 16 hours a day, leaving an eating window of 8 hours, is called the 16:8 method or the Leangains diet. During the 16:8 diet, men fast for 16 hours each day, and women fast for 14 hours. This type of intermittent fast may be helpful for someone who has already tried the 12-hour fast but did not see any benefits. On this fast, people usually finish their evening meal by 8 p.m. and then skip breakfast the next day, not eating again until noon.

A study on mice found that limiting the feeding window to 8 hours protected them from obesity, inflammation, diabetes, and liver disease, even when they ate the same total number of calories as mice that ate whenever they wished.

3. Fasting for 2 days a week

People following the 5:2 diet eat standard amounts of healthful food for 5 days and reduce calorie intake on the other 2 days. During the 2 fasting days, men generally consume 600 calories and women 500 calories. Typically, people separate their fasting days in the week. For example, they may fast on a Monday and Thursday and eat normally on the other days. There should be at least 1 non-fasting day between fasting days.

There is limited research on the 5:2 diet, which is also known as the Fast diet. A study involving 107 overweight or obese women found that restricting calories twice weekly and continuous calorie restriction both led to similar Fat loss. A small-scale study looked at the effects of this fasting style in 23 overweight women. Over the course of one menstrual cycle, the women lost 4.8 percent of their body weight and 8.0 percent of their total body fat. However, these measurements returned to normal for most of the women after 5 days of normal eating.

4. Alternate day fasting

There are several variations of the alternate day fasting plan, which involves fasting every other day. For some people, alternate day fasting means a complete avoidance of solid foods on fasting days, while other people allow up to 500 calories. On feeding days, people often choose to eat as much as they want.

One study reports that alternate day fasting is effective for Fat loss and heart health in both healthy and overweight adults. The researchers found that the 32 participants lost an average of 5.2 kilograms (kg), or just over 11 pounds (lb), over a 12-week period. Alternate day fasting is quite an extreme form of intermittent fasting, and it may not be suitable for beginners or those with certain medical conditions. It may also be difficult to maintain this type of fasting in the long term.

5. A weekly 24-hour fast

On a 24-hour diet, a person can have teas and calorie-free drinks. Fasting completely for 1 or 2 days a week, known as the Eat-Stop-Eat diet, involves eating no food for 24 hours at a time. Many people fast from breakfast to breakfast or lunch to lunch.

People on this diet plan can have water, tea, and other calorie-free drinks during the fasting period. People should return to normal eating patterns on the non-fasting days. Eating in this manner reduces a person's total calorie intake but does not limit the specific foods that the individual consumes.

A 24-hour fast can be challenging, and it may cause fatigue, headaches, or irritability. Many people find that these effects become less extreme over time as the body adjusts to this new pattern of eating. People may benefit from trying a 12-hour or 16-hour fast before transitioning to the 24-hour fast.

6. Meal skipping

This flexible approach to intermittent fasting may be good for beginners. It involves occasionally skipping meals.   People can decide which meals to skip according to their level of hunger or time restraints. However, it is important to eat healthful foods at each meal.

Meal skipping is likely to be most successful when individuals monitor and respond to their body's hunger signals. Essentially, people using this style of intermittent fasting will eat when they are hungry and skip meals when they are not. This may feel more natural for some people than the other fasting methods.

7. The Warrior Diet

The Warrior Diet is a relatively extreme form of intermittent fasting.

The Warrior Diet involves eating very little, usually just a few servings of raw fruit and vegetables, during a 20-hour fasting window, then eating one large meal at night. The eating window is usually only around 4 hours.

This form of fasting may be best for people who have tried other forms of intermittent fasting already. Supporters of the Warrior Diet claim that humans are natural nocturnal eaters and that eating at night allows the body to gain nutrients in line with its circadian rhythms. During the 4-hour eating phase, people should make sure that they consume plenty of vegetables, proteins, and healthful fats. They should also include some carbohydrates.

Although it is possible to eat some foods during the fasting period, it can be challenging to stick to the strict guidelines on when and what to eat in the long term. Also, some people struggle with eating such a large meal so close to bedtime. There is also a risk that people on this diet will not eat enough nutrients, such as fiber. This can increase the risk of cancer and have an adverse effect on digestive and immune health.

Tips for maintaining intermittent fasting

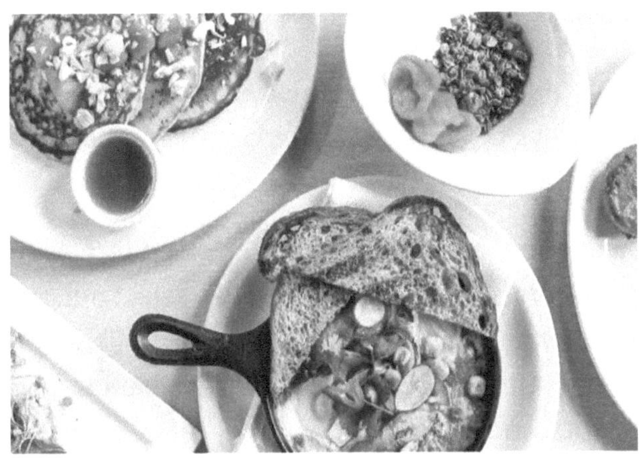

Yoga and light exercise may help to make intermittent fasting easier.

Yoga and light exercise may help to make intermittent fasting easier.

It can be challenging to stick to an intermittent fasting program.

The following tips may help people stay on track and maximize the benefits of intermittent fasting:

Staying hydrated. Drink lots of water and calorie-free drinks, such as herbal teas, throughout the day.

Avoiding obsessing over food. Plan plenty of distractions on fasting days to avoid thinking about food, such as catching up on paperwork or going to see a movie.

Resting and relaxing. Avoid strenuous activities on fasting days, although light exercise such as yoga may be beneficial.

Making every calorie count. If the chosen plan allows some calories during fasting periods, select nutrient-dense foods that are rich in protein, fiber, and healthful fats. Examples include beans, lentils, eggs, fish, nuts, and avocado.

Eating high-volume foods. Select filling yet low-calorie foods, which include popcorn, raw vegetables, and fruits with high water content, such as grapes and melon.

Increasing the taste without the calories. Season meals generously with garlic, herbs, spices, or vinegar. These foods are extremely low in calories yet are full of flavor, which may help to reduce feelings of hunger.

Choosing nutrient-dense foods after the fasting period. Eating foods that are high in fiber, vitamins, minerals, and other nutrients helps to keep blood sugar levels steady and prevent nutrient deficiencies. A balanced diet will also contribute to Fat loss and overall health.

There are many different ways to do intermittent fasting, and there is no single plan that will work for everyone. Individuals will experience the best results if they try out the various styles to see what suits their lifestyle and preferences.

Regardless of the type of intermittent fasting, fasting for extended periods when the body is unprepared can be problematic. These forms of dieting may not be suitable for everyone. If a person is prone to disordered eating, these approaches may exacerbate their unhealthy relationship with food.

People with health conditions, including diabetes, should speak to a doctor before attempting any form of fasting. For the best results, it is essential to eat a healthful and balanced diet on non-fasting days. If necessary, a person can seek professional help to personalize an intermittent fasting plan and avoid pitfalls.

CHAPTER EIGHT

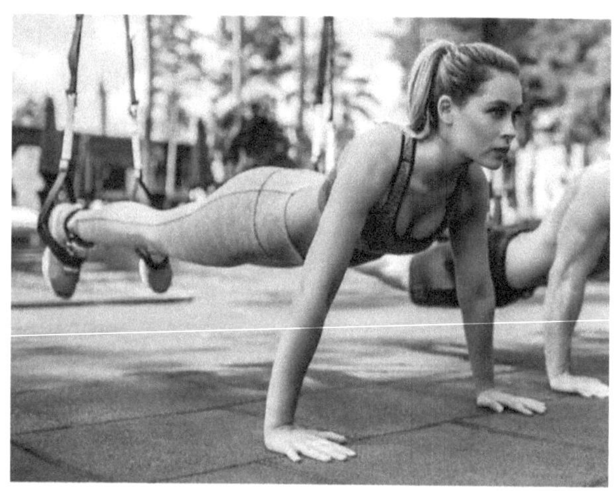

The Best Exercise to Lose Fat - It is Amazing How These Simple Exercises Will Make You Shed Fat Fast

One of the main reasons why people exercise is to lose fat. Therefore, they tend to search for best exercises to lose fat. Diet alone will not give you optimum results. That is the reason why you need to couple it with exercise. Below are the ways you can exercise and lose fat.

1 - Combined strength and aerobic exercise. When you are choosing your work-outs, consider cross training to significantly reduce fat in your body.

2 - Weight lifting. You can go to your local gym and ask for their weight lifting facility. This can be one of the best exercises to lose fat as well as tone your muscles.

3 - Work out on different muscle group each day. Basically, muscles need to recuperate within 48 hours after working out to avoid muscle straining and overstretching. If you worked on your legs today, you can work on your arms tomorrow.

4 - Cardio exercises. Always include cardio exercises in your routine. This will let you burn fat and eventually lose them. Do this in at least 3 times for every week.

5 - Go for a jog. Go for exercises that will keep you motivated, fun and easy to do. Jogging is one easy exercise you can do everyday to keep you occupied and physically active.

When you exercise, your heart will pump more blood. Therefore, this increases release of oxygen into your muscles as well as increase your metabolism. Once your body increases its metabolism, it will burn fat contents as a source of the energy during the process. Exercise not only to lose fat but to gain long term benefits as well.

Best Time of Day to Work Out

Finding time to exercise can be challenging, and the most important thing is to squeeze in any amount of it whenever you can. But if you want to optimize your workouts to get the widest range of benefits, you might want to try exercising in the morning.

Here's what the science says about the best time of day to exercise — and what to expect if you opt for later workouts.

Morning workouts have an edge

Working out in the morning — especially on an empty stomach — is the best way to burn stored fat, making it ideal for Fat loss. That's largely because the body's hormonal composition in the morning is set up to support that goal, says Anthony Hackney, a professor in the department of exercise and sport science at the University of North Carolina Chapel Hill.

In the early morning hours, you have a hormonal profile that would predispose you to better metabolism of fat. People naturally have elevated levels of cortisol and growth hormone in the morning—both of which are involved in metabolism—so you'll draw more of your energy from your fat reserves. That can potentially help with Fat loss. Research also suggests that morning exercisers may have less of an appetite throughout the day, which could also help protect them from putting on pounds.

Even if you hate early alarms, working out first thing in the morning can quickly become second nature. A study recently published in the Journal of Physiology found that exercising at 7 a.m. may shift your body clock earlier, meaning you'll feel more alert in the morning and get tired earlier in the evening, potentially priming you to get enough rest to wake up and do the same thing the next day. Some research even suggests that it's easier to stick to healthy habits completed in the morning.

A morning sweat may also lead to better mental health and productivity throughout the day, since exercise is great for reducing stress. But if you're really not a morning person, don't force it. You may be exercising, but it may be at such a low intensity level that you're really not expending a lot of energy.

Afternoon workouts are almost as good

If you can swing a lunchtime workout, Afternoon workout is not a bad second choice — especially if you're trying to do a very long or rigorous routine.

Morning workouts are ideal for burning fat and losing weight, but afternoon workouts may give your performance a boost, since you'll have eaten a meal or two by the time you get going. Any time you eat, your blood sugar levels rise. Sugar in the form of blood glucose is one of the things we need if we're trying to work at a higher intensity.

An afternoon workout can also be a great way to avoid an end-of-the-day slump. The Journal of Physiology study found that exercising between 1 p.m. and 4 p.m. can shift forward your body clock in the same way as an early morning workout. Even taking a quick walk may help you perk up and refocus.

One preliminary paper from 2018 found that your body naturally burns about 10% more calories in the late afternoon, compared to the early morning and late night. The researchers looked at bodies at rest — so they can't draw firm conclusions about what happens when people work out — but it's possible that you could burn a little extra energy if you move in the afternoon.

Night time workouts still come with perks

For many people, exercising is most convenient after work. But there's a common belief that evening exercise perks you up so much that it's difficult to fall asleep later.

While the Journal of Physiology study found that exercising between 7 p.m. and 10 p.m. delays the body clock, translating to later bedtimes, Evidence suggests that, as long as you're not exercising, showering and then [immediately] jumping in bed to go to sleep, it doesn't interfere with your sleep pattern at all. A stress-relieving activity like yoga may even help you sleep better if it's done at night.

And while the research about morning workouts and Fat loss is more established, some evidence suggests that nighttime workouts can also set people up for Fat loss. A new paper published in the journal Experimental Physiology found that nighttime workouts do not disrupt sleep, and over time can also reduce levels of the hunger-stimulating hormone ghrelin, which could help with Fat loss or management.

If he had to pick a best time to exercise, morning would win. Early workouts make the most of your biology and psychology, potentially leading to better results and adherence over time. But there's really no bad time to exercise, Hackney reiterates, and the most important thing is finding the time to do so, whenever works for you.

If you will do it in the morning, do it. If you will do it in the evening, do it. "If your physiology is not going to match up with your behavior, then it's a moot point.

10 Effective Morning Exercises for Fat loss

Do you know it is best to work out in the morning? The best thing you can add to your workout regime is an AM workout. The busy, minute-by-minute lives we lead nowadays have just messed up our entire natural system. Workouts have always been meant for the mornings. Ayurvedic Dincharya (which I suggest to all pretty ladies to incorporate in your lives; trust me it works wonders!) puts Vyayama (exercise) right after cleansing of the senses.

Why Should We Work Out In Mornings?

It keeps our body healthy. It also helps to eliminate toxins from the body that have built up and accumulated overnight.

It rejuvenates and recharges our body, gearing it up for maximum performance. Studies show that people who exercise in the morning burn up a higher percentage of fat. Exercising in the morning increases our core temperature for the rest of the day. That means that you not only burn fat during your workout but also throughout the day. When we do something early in the day, we are more likely to be consistent about it as nothing can come between us and our fitness goals. Right?

What Should My AM Workout Comprise Of?

Your morning workout routine to lose weight could be anything starting from running to swimming, dancing, skipping, HIITs, jogging, walking, anything! It is all about that as a fit girl what do you feel like doing that morning. But for those trying to lose weight, you have to be a little more concerned about what will burn off the most calories and how. So here is a guide to your AM workout for Fat loss.

Cardio:

Cardio exercises are the most important when one is trying to lose weight. The first step to Fat loss is burning calories, right? It is a fact that doing cardio first thing in the morning, on an empty stomach, helps your muscles to oxidize the accumulated fatty acids in the body. In simple words, you will burn the stored fat off the body and not the calories that you have just consumed.

Here is given 10 best cardio exercises to do in the morning, which in turn will help you to lose weight for a healthy and fit body.

1. Go for a Run or Walk:

Though you can run on the treadmill, try going outside as the fresh air, free from pollution provides good things for your heart, lungs and mind. It helps you to connect with nature.

2. Biking:

This is another cardio exercise to burn calories. Biking helps not only to burn calories but also gives effective endurance training to those leg muscles. While running affects mainly your calf muscles and shins, biking works well for the thighs. You can vary your speed between normal and all-out. It helps in building endurance. It is best to go for cycling in the morning to avoid traffic.

3. Circuit Training:

This is another cardio exercise to burn calories. Biking helps not only to burn calories but also gives effective endurance training to those leg muscles. While running affects mainly your calf muscles and shins, biking works well for the thighs. You can vary your speed between normal and all-out. It helps in building endurance. It is best to go for cycling in the morning to avoid traffic.

It is basically a form of body conditioning that targets strength building and muscle endurance through high intensity aerobics. The idea is to do all the exercises that complete one circuit and then repeat the circuit again, taking time only to sip water between the circuits. There are many circuit examples available in the form of DVDs and YouTube videos. Personally I like doing the Jillian Michaels' DVD for circuit training, cardio videos of Cassey Ho and the workouts by Bob Harper, all available on YouTube. Some of my favorite exercises for circuit training are burpees, squat jumps, plank lifts, and hand walks. Circuit training burns 30 percent extra calories than normal workouts. Mornings are the best time to do circuits as you are full of energy to put all of it into the exercise. This will help to burn those calories away.

4. Kickboxing:

Training for kickboxing is beneficial enough to make you stronger. It also burns fat and gives you real good moves to use in self-defense. There are many fun kickboxing workouts available online. It is best to join a kickboxing class for initial training. This is one of the best morning exercise for Fat loss.

5. Yoga:

It is a known fact that the best and also the most appropriate time to do yoga asanas is in the morning, preferably before or at the time of sunrise. It should always be done on an empty stomach. Practicing yoga not only tones the body externally but also helps in the healing and strengthening of the internal organs.

6. Surya Namaskar:

A single Surya Namaskar burns 13.91 calories approx. If you practice Surya Namaskar for 30 minutes in the morning and complete about 15 rounds, you burn nearly about 278-280 calories. This is more than what one normally might burn during a 1 hour cardio session. As there are many versions of Surya Namaskar to suit one's fitness level, choose one for yourself. Surya Namaskar is suggested to be performed at the time of sunrise. It is not only about burning calories but also about the overall well-being of a person. Try to complete as many Surya Namaskar as possible. Do not overburden yourself at one go. Start with 6 or 8 SN, and keep increasing the number as you get comfortable.

7. Stretching Exercises:

Stretching exercises are a must in your daily routine. Even on your rest-days, do try a few nice stretching exercises. Studies suggest that overnight proteins get collected in the joints. It is important to stretch your muscles and work your joints to prevent diseases like arthritis. Further, these stretching exercises tone your muscles. It is important to add toning to your workout regime. After burning the calories, it comes to toning it all up. Yogasanas like Downward-Dog, Cobra, Virasana variations and Cat-stretch combine toning and stretching.

8. Pranayama:

It has been a long time since Yoga guru Baba Ramdev popularized Pranayama among the masses, and it is still a craze. Pranayama has the power to keep you fit and young. This too must be practiced on an empty stomach.

9. Kapalbhati Pranayama:

It is one cure for everything and one of the simplest techniques to deal with all types of diseases. It helps to lose fat from the stomach area (the most stubborn fat too). If you are a beginner, do this exercise for 3 minutes and then keep progressing up to 10 minutes. That is the maximum limit for Kapalbhati. The ideal way is to do 700 counts of Kapalbhati every day.

10. Nadi Pranayama or Anulom-Vilom:

Nadi Pranayama or Anulom-Vilom is another common Pranayama which can be done by anyone from a little child to your 80-year old grandma. The most important thing about Anulom-Vilom is that it helps in regulating breathing. The breathing technique is important during all kinds of exercises, especially while doing cardio and yoga. This can affect your Fat loss and toning. Breathing exercises forms an important part of Anulom-Vilom.

Conclusion

It is good to do your AM cardio workout on an empty stomach. Make sure you stay hydrated all the time! You can use water, infused water, coconut water, whichever you find healthy.

If you are doing weight training after your cardio sessions, make sure you grab some protein beforehand like a banana or some almonds.

Try doing Abhyanga (self-massage with oil) before your morning workout. It is an Ayurvedic ritual that helps in the removal of toxins and keeps your body moisturized throughout the workout.

Since your beauty is as important as your fitness, make sure to apply sunscreen lotion if you are heading outside for a run or biking.

www.ingramcontent.com/pod-product-compliance
Lightning Source LLC
Chambersburg PA
CBHW051213250726

48655CB00006B/2386